I0453846

Hemicrania

Copyright © 2024 by Therese Gleason

Cover image by Sheila Gomes
Author's Photo by Katheryn Costello
Edited by Maria S. Picone
Cover design by James Rawlings and Teresa Snow

All rights reserved. No part of this publication may be reproduced, distributed or transmitted in any form or by any means, including photocopying, recording, or other electronic or mechanical methods, without the prior written permission of the publisher, except in the case of brief quotations embodied in critical reviews and certain other noncommercial uses permitted by copyright law. For permission requests, write to the publisher at the email address below.

Chestnut Review Chapbooks, an imprint of Chestnut Review LLC
Ithaca, New York
https://chestnutreview.com
ISBN: 978-1-965158-07-4

In *Hemicrania*, poet Therese Gleason reaches out through the "half-headed pain" of the migraineur, despite (or rather, because of) "her head a cracked bell/ that wouldn't stop ringing." Like the two halves of the brain, this chapbook succeeds by dualities. Both thematically cohesive and formally expansive, *Hemicrania* tells the story, on one side, of the mostly male failures of medicine, and on the other, of the matrilineal inheritance of suffering "which women must endure." Borrowing language from medicine but wholly rooted in poetry, the Patient is both reduced to the base elements of piss, salt, bile, and snot and elevated to the mystic, ghostly realm of saints, incantation, and prayer. Gleason asks "what angel, message, lesson" can be found in suffering. But even if, in the end, the Patient resigns, "I'm no more chosen than I am god/forsaken," the poet has made from her suffering this simultaneously delicate and explosive contribution to the literature of women's chronic pain.

—Cynthia Marie Hoffman, author of *Exploding Head*

Chronic and episodic migraine patients will agree that they'll do anything and everything to exorcise the migraine demon. Author Therese Gleason attempts just that in *Hemicrania* via revelatory poems brimming with prayers, incantations, and supplications. The poet gives readers the 4-1-1 from the front lines of Migrainesville in poems that confront medical sexism and medical gaslighting—and in poems that explore the conundrum of genetic inheritance. The vulnerability and daily struggle of the person with migraine are depicted with vivid accuracy and candor. *Hemicrania* should reside on the nightstands of poetry lovers, patients, physicians, and caregivers.

—Rita Maria Martinez, author of *The Jane and Bertha in Me*

To read *Hemicrania* is to witness a poet contend with profound spiritual and physical agony. In found poems, hybrid forms, and collages, Gleason traces her family's matrilineal inheritance of migraine alongside an enraging genealogy of the medical establishment's all-too-frequent disregard for migraineurs' suffering. And while *Hemicrania* is a scorching account of migraine's brutal toll on body and mind, in its pages Gleason offers too a psalter of companionship: invocations, incantations, and charms against pain drawn from a thousand years of belief and experience. The unflinching intimacy of these poems humbled me.

—Carolyn Oliver, author of *Inside the Storm I Want to Touch the Tremble*

In *Hemicrania*, a gut-wrenching and aesthetically innovative portrait of the matrilineal curse of migraine, Therese Gleason renders the ineffable. Equal parts masterclass in vivifying the medical archive and gripping reportage from the patient's vantage, Gleason's intimate poems shatter migraineurs' isolation to deliver spells for a painless future.

—Sarah M. Sala, author of *Devil's Lake*

Hemicrania

Therese Gleason

Chestnut Review Chapbooks

For my mother, my grandmothers, my daughters,
and migraineurs everywhere

Contents

Annunciation 1

Self-Portrait as Barometer 2

Migraine Disability Assessment Test 1 3

Our Lady of the Burning Bush 4

Headache Charm 5

Aura 7

Cortical Spreading Depression 8

Revenant 9

In Her/My Head 10

Migraineur 16

Remedia 18

Prayer for the Intercession of Saint Teresa of Ávila, Patron
    Saint of Migraines 19

Photophobia 20

A Kind of Brainstorm 21

On the Heredity of Migraine 22

MRI 23

In Bed 24

Migraine Abecedarian 26

Maiden, Mother, Crone 28

Headache Stone 29

Incantation 30

Self-Portrait as Warming Planet 31

Mums 32

The Fathers of Modern Headache Medicine Discuss the
    Migrainous Woman and All Her Troubles 34

Migraine Disability Assessment Test Redux 36

Faith Healing 37

Postdrome 38

Ode to the Jaw 39

Self-Portrait at 45, on the Autumnal Equinox 40

Notes 42

Acknowledgments 47

About the Author 49

Annunciation

Always the gray dawn
when the pain angel appears:
strange bells ring in my ears,
tinkling up and down my limbs.
I dissipate into the bruised
half-moons under my eyes.
The sun's white light glares
on the horizon—it must be almost five.

On the bathroom floor,
I think of Mary, who said *Behold*:
I am the handmaid of the Lord,
let it be done to me…
but I would pass this chalice if I could—
and I have, to my daughters.
My mother to me, her mother
to her: a trinity of Marys,
none of us unscathed.

Agony makes me crave
meaning, not just relief.
I want to commune with martyrs,
sweat blood, trade in miracles
or a little holiness, at least.
But even with my head
exploding, I know the truth:
I'm no more chosen than I'm god
forsaken.

Self-Portrait as Barometer

I knew it would rain today
by the ache in my left temple
that woke me at dawn,
before the sky went violet:
a herd of thunderheads
stomping till musty petrichor
seeped up from the earth's cellar
and leaves twisted
in the corkscrew wind.

I was born in tornado alley,
brain primed to sense fronts—
a sudden coldness on the breeze,
a tone of voice trending sharp
or flat, my mother's clenched
jaw, hand on her hip.
I grew skilled at predicting weather
but never could control it—
I sheltered in the basement,
where I drew yellow suns
and blue skies in chalk
on cinderblock walls.

Migraine Disability Assessment Test 1

And I am constantly fettered by sickness, and often in the grip of pain so intense that it threatens to kill me...

—Hildegard of Bingen (c. 1175)

The Migraine Disability Assessment Test

██ measure the impact ██
headaches have on your life ██ inform ████████████████████████ care ████
deter ████████████ pain and disability ████████████████ find ████ treatment ████

INSTRUCTIONS

████████████████████████ about ALL of the headaches you have had ████████
████████████████████████████ your health ████████████

_____ 1. ████ many days ████████████ you miss work or school because of ██ headache ██

_____ 2. ██ many days ████████████ productivity ████████ reduced ████████
because of ██ headache ██ Do ████████ you count ████████████████
████

_____ 3. ██ many days ████████████ no ████████████████████████
caring for children ████ because of ██ headaches ██

_____ 4. ██ many days ████████████████████████████████
██ of ██ headache ████████████ you counted ████████████ you did not do
house ██ work ██

_____ 5. ██ many days ████████████ you miss family ████████████ because of ██
headaches ██

_____ Total (Questions 1-5)

What your Physician will need to know about your headache:

_____ A. ████ many days ████████████ you have a headache ████████████ more than 1
██ count each day ██

_____ B. ████████████████████ painful ██████ headaches ██████ pain ████████
pain ██ bad as it can be ██

Scoring: After you have filled out this questionnaire, add the total number of days from questions 1-5 (ignore A and B).

MIDAS Grade	Definition	MIDAS Score
I	Little or No Disability	0-5
II	Mild Disability	6-10
III	Moderate Disability	11-20
IV	Severe Disability	21+

If Your MIDAS Score is 6 or more, please discuss this with your doctor.

Our Lady of the Burning Bush

And the angel of the Lord appeared unto him in flame of fire
out of the midst of a bush: and he looked, and, behold, the
bush burned with fire, and the bush was not consumed.

—Exodus, 3:2

Lizard brain shakes awake before dawn,
stumbling for pills and ice, too late—wildfire
spreads, engulfs my head. I pace, repose
unbearable. Hot and cold sweat blooming,
guttural urgency. On my knees, I retch
so hard I piss myself, expelling salt,
bile, snot. Teeth clattering, spittle dangles
from my chin. Cranial crescendo: pain
peaks, recedes. Euphoric, I'm scoured, wrung,
almost holy with relief, a vessel—
what angel, message, lesson? But the trickster
body balks. I slump, the brutal throb builds.
I'm no saint but this feels like a test:
O, *kyrie*, may this pain purify me.

Headache Charm

Walk toward horizon
at low tide

>   to gather sand dollars
>   pungent with brine.

Hum a lullaby, waves
lapping your feet.

>   Collect tears in the cup
>   of a scallop shell:

open palm ridged
like newly cut teeth.

>   Take three sips
>   of saltwater wine,

holy water
from body's sea.

>   Place a cake urchin
>   under your tongue

and crown your skull
with seaweed wreath.

>   Make an offering
>   to the pain angel:

mermaid coins
brown and furred,

not yet bleached.
Lie down on the beach,

a cockle shell
over each eye.

Count backwards
from infinity.

Aura

Tonight, a **pale** disc
shrouded in gauze passes overhead

like the **moon** in disguise.
I walk the dog around the block,

past the **strobing** streetlight
that vexes my **brain**.

It's been flashing like an **emergency** for days.
I keep thinking I should **call** someone—

the city, my mother, **God?**
Swaths of mist and dim greenish haze

drift over **pinprick** stars
sunk deep in the **sockets** of the sky—

I **blink**, rubbing my eyes:
for a **flashbulb** second

I'm blind.

Cortical Spreading Depression

A shower * of sparks * *

```
    *   *              *
    *                  *
    *                  *


*              **               *
```

signals the event horizon:

```
(      ********************      )
```

a black hole
```
*********
*********
*********
```

yawning behind

```
***      ***
***      ***
***      ***
```

my eye.

(*)

Revenant

Seized by a ghost, the temple gets sick. Seized by a ghost, the temple is wretched.
Seized by a ghost, the head is sick and wretched.

—Incantation against headache, Nineveh, 7th c. B.C.E.

The woman in the white night
gown came for me,

tendrils lank like snakes
plastering her gray face.

She didn't talk, just hummed,
head in her hands.

She came just before sunrise
& I knew she wanted to stick

a bony finger through my eye
until my body jerked

like a witch in a noose
& my guts churned,

extremities prickling,
crown ablaze.

In Her/My Head

Urgent Care, August 2021

English, which can express the thoughts of Hamlet and the tragedy of Lear, has no words for the shiver and the headache…let a sufferer try to describe a pain in his head to a doctor and language at once runs dry.

—Virginia Woolf, "On Being Ill" (1926)

CHIEF COMPLAINT
45-year-old female patient presented with severe nausea, vomiting associated with typical migraines probably triggered by a tension headache.
DESCRIPTION OF HEADACHES
Patient woke up at 4 AM this morning with severe migraine and also nausea, vomiting and has not been able to keep anything down. Location of pain: *bilateral* Character of pain: *throbbing* Severity of pain: *severe* Accompanying symptoms: *photophobia*
DEGREE OF FUNCTIONAL IMPAIRMENT
Moderate

45 year-old female Patient
presented at clinic a gray-faced ghost,
her head a cracked bell
that wouldn't stop ringing,
guts hollow and wrung.

Patient, shaky and parched,
not allowed to enter,
(throwing up a symptom of Covid),
told to wait outside
clutching a plastic bag of her own sick
Never mind that her neurologist
had called ahead, prescribing
IV fluids and meds.

In tears, still vomiting up nothing
but air, bile, and spit,
Patient gave up.
Better to sip Gatorade in bed
than wait in her car in the bright
sun and heat with nothing to drink.

CURRENT USE OF MEDS TO TREAT HA
Abortive meds? *Imitrex* Prophylactic Med: *no; patient has tried and failed riboflavin, magnesium, Sumatriptan, Treximet, Rizatriptan, and beta-blocker I recommended due to history of bronchial allergy. Has not tried Tricyclic or Topamax.*

PHYSICAL EXAM
General: *awake, alert, oriented, in no acute distress*

PLAN
• *Metoclopramide HCl (REGLAN) 5 MG/ML injection* • *Diphenhydramine (BENADRYL) 50 MG/ML injection* • *Sodium Chloride (NaCl) 0.9 % solution*

Back home, Patient tried an alternate route
inserting a suppository
since her body had refused
all capsules and tablets,
even the one that melted
under her tongue like a communion wafer.
Patient got into a hot bath
with ice behind her neck
to draw the pain from her head
down through her feet.
She tried prayer and sleep
but was forsaken.

Patient's husband drove her back to Urgent Care
an hour before closing.
Patient made to wait outside again
till darkness fell
and Doctor let her in through the back—
in case her migraine
was contagious.
Hair matted, face a death mask,
Patient dug deep to extract language
from her malfunctioning brain.
Explained she'd lost count after 15
but had been vomiting from dawn to dusk,
had tried all her pills, charms, and tricks
but the migraine wouldn't quit.

Doctor asked Patient if she had Pedialyte,
said he'd like to give her an injection
with the migraine cocktail
but not the IV
because *the drip takes time*
and *I'd hate to keep my nurses here late.*
Patient tried to insist
but ended up begging.

PROGRESS NOTES

Patient follow-up better
after liter of IV normal saline
with 5 mg Metoclopramide
and 25mg Diphenhydramine.

I told her that if the headache comes back
she can also use 600 Ibuprofen
and also the rectal Compazine
given by neurology.

INSTRUCTIONS

We discussed extensively about stress
management since I think
this is a huge trigger for her migraines
and possible tension headache
and the patient was very receptive
to the message and resources
(Take the stress out of your life
by Jay Winner, MD; Palouse Mindfulness;
YouTube: "Stress Management
with Dr. L___"; Interviews of the Dalai Lama
and Archbishop Desmond Tutu)
that I gave her.

Nurse came and was brisk,
didn't check on Patient or offer a blanket
when she started to shiver,
forgot to unhook Patient
from the IV when it stopped, timer beeping.
Patient wheeled her IV cart into the hallway,
dark red blood filling
the clear tube taped to her arm,
to flag an orderly.
Patient had been awake for 20 hours
and was shaking from the Reglan
in the cold saline drip.

Doctor returned, apologized
for *rushing her* at first,
said he liked to take his time.
Patient wanted to slump in the seat
of her husband's car waiting
in the parking lot
but now Doctor
had all the time in the world for her.
Doctor told Patient to read
The Book of Joy and try meditation.
Jaw clenched, Patient couldn't find
the words, the strength
to get up and walk out.
Patient seethed
but thanked Doctor anyway.
Even now, Patient's still shaking
her head,
shaking off blame
and shame.

(text on left from doctor's after-visit summary, notes, and discharge instructions recorded in online MyChart)

Migraineur

I have cradled three generations of heads in my palms,
        temples racked with grief: my mother's,
                my daughter's, my own.

It begins with a whiff of danger, heat
        & chill shimmering.
                Dread tightens my gut

& pain sharpens from throb to hot poker,
        eclipsing my vision. I scramble for pills,
                willing my body to absorb the medicine,

abort the storm. Lights out, I close the bedroom door
        on my life, ice pack at the back
                of my neck, pillow bruising scalp.

Nausea rises & I race to the toilet
        to retch till relief breaks out
                on my brow. I sink to the floor,

face down on cool tile, where I stay, heaving bile & air
        in 20-minute intervals. Salt slicks my skin,
                seeps from my eyes, nose & throat.

Face washed gray as agony
        encircles my cranium, I remember
                tiptoeing to place a wet washcloth

over my mother's eyes as she lay moaning, saltines
        & warm Coke untouched;
                coming home from school to tangled sheets,

her hooked to an IV in the hospital, again & I wonder
        what drives this malady afflicting
                my maternal line, not the physical triggers—

weather, hormones, hunger, thirst—but psychic sources
        carried forward in the souls of cells
                that remember fractured attachments

stashed in the darkest corners of the root cellar,
        reverberating in my blood today:
                legacy that courses through my daughter's

shuddering body as saltwater & drugs weep
        from a plastic bag into her vein.
                I hold her small hand, paralyzed

like my great-grandmother—whose attacks
        froze half her body—powerless
                to stop the pain.

Remedia

Bald's *Leechbook*, c. 950 C.E.

For ache of half the head
take the red nettle of one stalk,
bruise it, mingle with vinegar
and the white of an egg,
put all together, anoint therewith.
For a half heads ache, bruise
in vinegar with oil the clusters
of the laurus, smear the cheek with that.
For the same, take juice of rue, wring
on the nostril which is on the sore side.
For a half heads ache, take dust
of the clusters of laurel, and mustard,
mingle them together, pour vinegar
upon them, smear with that
on the sore side. Or mix with wine
the clusters of laurel. Or rub fine
in vinegar the seed of rue,
put equal quantities of both,
rub the back of the neck...

Prayer for the Intercession of Saint Teresa of Ávila, Patron Saint of Migraines

O namesake saint
of visions and ecstasy,
pray for me—
death dogged
and bone bleeding.

I will boil *wild Dasye roots*
with a dozen greate earthewormes
and eat them or pound them
to smear across my face.
I will say 100 Our Fathers
and 200 Hail Marys—

Photophobia

In a dark time, the eye begins to see...

—Theodore Roethke

Vampiric, I shun the sun:

the flesh-eating rays
carved a hole in my nose.

I crave shade, night, the grave

dark—cool marsupial pockets.
Yellow glare ignites

a pupillary bruise, sonar rippling

to my brain, temple, cathedral of pain—
the migraine's holy see.

Who needs light—or sight?

In Mammoth Cave
fish glide through the Mystic:

finned tongues, pink-white, eye-

less, sensory papillae
their underwater guides.

A Kind of Brainstorm

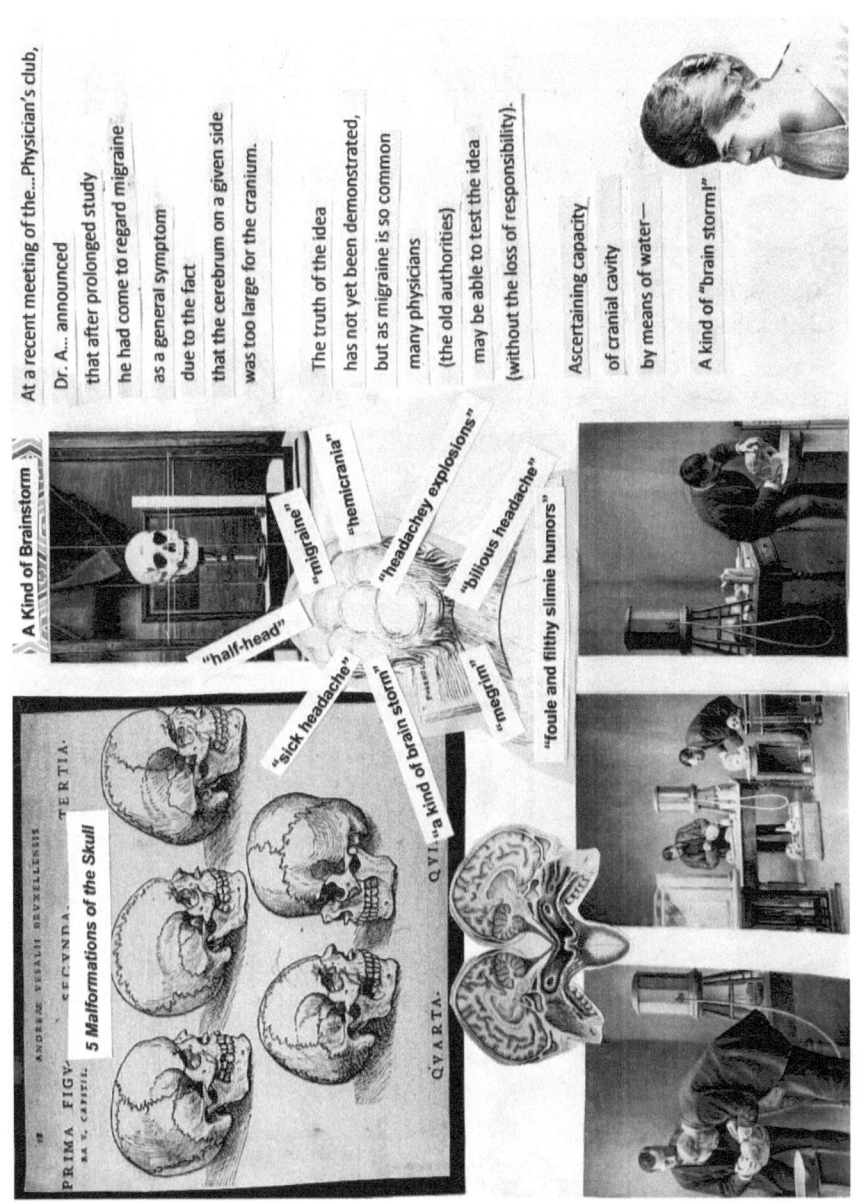

> A Kind of Brainstorm :

At a recent meeting of the...Physician's club,

Dr. A... announced

that after prolonged study

he had come to regard migraine

as a general symptom

due to the fact

that the cerebrum on a given side

was too large for the cranium.

The truth of the idea

has not yet been demonstrated,

but as migraine is so common

many physicians

(the old authorities)

may be able to test the idea

(without the loss of responsibility).

Ascertaining capacity

of cranial cavity

by means of water—

A kind of "brain storm!"

"migraine"

"hemicrania"

"half-head"

"headachey explosions"

"bilious headache"

"sick headache"

"a kind of brain storm"

"megrim"

"foule and filthy slimie humors"

5 Malformations of the Skull

PRIMA FIGV. SECVNDA. TERTIA.

QVARTA. QVI.

ANDREAE VESALII BRVXELLENSIS

On the Heredity of Migraine

—from the 1920's newspaper columns of Dr. William Brady,
"Noted Physician and Author"

An unstable or vulnerable nervous system is inherited,
and on such a nervous system the effect of factors
which would not greatly upset a sound or stable nervous

system is expressed in various ways—epilepsy, hysteria,
neurasthenia (whatever that may be), alcoholism,
drug habits, cultism, and outright lunacy. Epilepsy

has been called a motor neurosis and migraine a sensory
neurosis. There is considerable similarity
between the two. Either condition is likely to occur

in the family of an alcoholic forbear or a feeble-minded
forbear or a drug addict or one who was "queer"
or frankly subject to one or another form of insanity.

But migraine, like epilepsy, may occur here and there
in a family where no such neurotic ancestry
can be traced. Does that sound discouraging? It shouldn't.

So precious few of us are blessed with an unstigmatized
inheritance! There are blots on every escutcheon.
But heredity is only one part: environment, education,

morality or ethics, and faith are the other four-fifths.

MRI

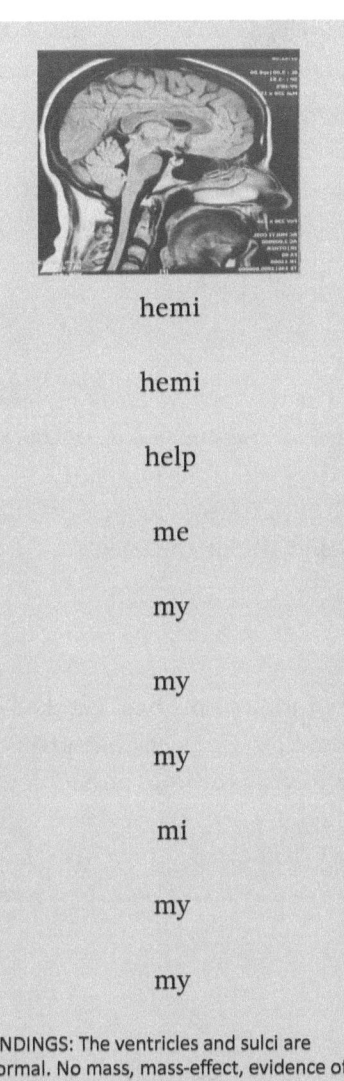

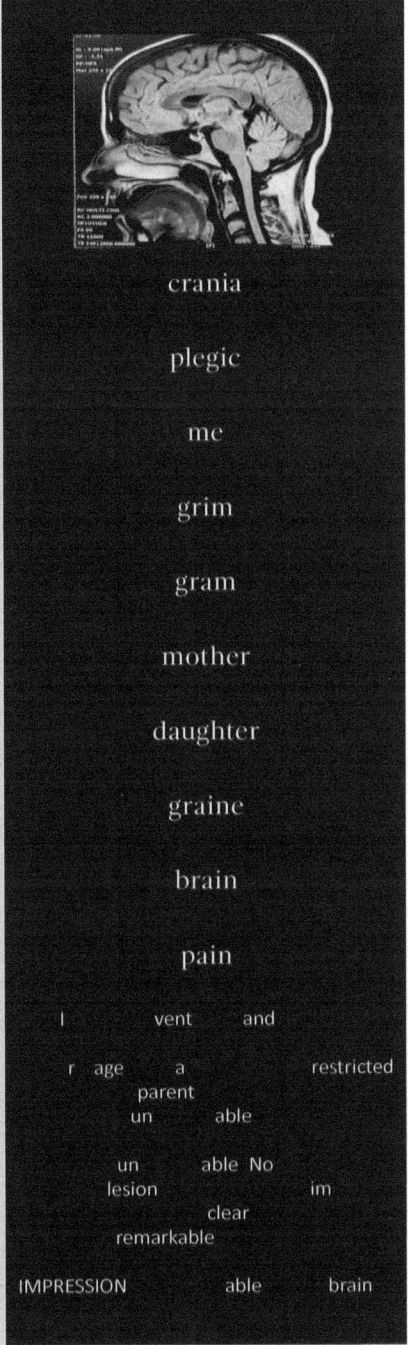

hemi	crania
hemi	plegic
help	me
me	grim
my	gram
my	mother
my	daughter
mi	graine
my	brain
my	pain

FINDINGS: The ventricles and sulci are normal. No mass, mass-effect, evidence of hemorrhage or infarct is seen. No restricted diffusion is apparent. The posterior fossa contents are unremarkable. Major arterial structures and dural venous sinuses are patent and unremarkable. No calvarial or skull base lesion is identified. The imaged paranasal sinuses are clear. The mastoid air cells are unremarkable

IMPRESSION: Unremarkable MRI of brain without contrast.

I vent and
r age a restricted
parent
un able
un able No
lesion im
clear
remarkable

IMPRESSION able brain

In Bed

Three, four, sometimes five times a month, I spend the day in bed with migraine headaches, insensible to the world around me. Almost every day of every month, between these attacks, I feel the sudden irrational irritation and the flush of blood into the cerebral arteries which tell me that a migraine is on its way, and I take certain drugs to avert its arrival. If I did not take the drugs, I would be able to function perhaps one day in four.

—Joan Didion, "In Bed" (1968)

When does episodic become chronic? The doctor says *fifteen or more headache days a month with three or more migraine symptoms for at least three months.* What about fourteen headache days with four migraine symptoms? What's worse: a month with seven severe migraines, or a month with thirty-one days of 'mild' pain without a break?

***

I worry my children will remember how I took to my bed, checked out of life. How many missed basketball games, track meets, birthdays, movie nights, dinners? Fifteen requests to walk the dog, turned down. Twelve pleas for homework help, declined. I worry my husband will get sick and tired of me being sick and tired. Too often, I turn over in bed, away—*I'm sorry, my head hurts. I don't want to have sex, or hear about your day.*

***

I've pushed through for years: lying on my office floor, door closed, eyes closed, praying the pills work before my hourlong commute; stumbling for ice in a hotel hallway on a business trip; vomiting, head in my hands, after staring at Zoom all day; teaching kindergarteners with the half-headed pain beaten back to a dull but insistent ache, little voices shrill bells, classroom windows without shades.

***

It's not that bad, I used to say. Not like my mother, who threw up blood and needed an IV—but now that's me, clutching a plastic shopping bag—bile, dark green—into which I've heaved, pulling over twice on the way to the ER, reassuring my kids I'll be ok.

***

Is it working? Is it working yet? my husband, my children, my friends, ask. I want to say *yes, yes, I feel so much better now.* But I don't know, and I'm afraid to disappoint them. To get my hopes up, again.

Migraine Abecedarian

I.

Acceptance and commitment therapy, acupuncture, Advil, Aimovig (preventive monthly shot), Aleve, Allegra, allergy shots, Aspartame avoidance (no diet drinks or Nutrasweet), Aspirin, Ayurveda, bargaining with God, bedrest, ~~Beta Blockers~~ (blood pressure too low), biofeedback, ~~birth control pills~~ (made headaches worse), Botox (in forehead, temples, scalp, and neck), caffeine (total avoidance/regular dosing–nothing in between), calling in sick (again), Calm app, chiropractic, Codeine, Coke (the drink, not the drug, although Freud took Cocaine for his), coffee, Compazine suppository (anti-emetic), counseling, craniosacral therapy, dairy-free, darkness, denial, driving myself to the ER with a barf bag, earplugs, energy healing, exercise, Fioricet (butalbital, acetaminophen, and caffeine), Flonase, ginger ale, gluten-free diet, hot bath with ice pack at back of neck, hot shower, ice, Imitrex (Sumatriptan), intravenous migraine cocktail (Reglan, Benadryl, Toradol, Triptan), IV saline (one bag for dehydration), jogging, kinesiology, kneading temples, lavender oil, lights out, lying face-down on cold bathroom tile, massage, Maxalt (orally disintegrating Rizatriptan Benzoate), menopause (jury's still out; my mom's lessened in frequency but didn't go away); mindfulness meditation, MRI (nothing wrong), Nasonex, no chocolate, no alcohol, no cheese, Nurtec (Calcitonin Gene Related Peptide receptor antagonist), night guard to prevent clenching, ~~NTI-tss~~ (dental device clipped on top front teeth; had to quit using so I wouldn't swallow in my sleep), orgasm, peppermint tea, Phenergan (suppository to quell nausea and bring on sleep), physical therapy, Pilates, pissing off coworkers by asking them not to wear perfume or cologne, prayer, pregnancy (daily headache during first trimester), physical therapy, Qi Gong, quiet, quitting jobs, quitting the gym, Reiki, Relpax (Eletriptan), silence, sleep, sleep study ("narcolepsoid" tendencies; invalid daytime sleepiness test—couldn't forgo caffeine), sunglasses, Tai Chi, ~~Topamax~~ (aka "Dopamax"), Transcendental Meditation, ~~Treximet~~ (Imitrex and Naproxen Sodium; insurance won't cover), Tylenol, ~~Ubrelvy~~ (insurance won't cover), undoing hairbands, unscented products (soap, shampoo, lotion, detergent), veganism, vegetarianism, vomiting, walking, whole foods diet, X-rays (nothing wrong), yoga, Zofran (anti-emetic), Zoloft (antidepressant), Zonisamide (anti-seizure), Zyrtec (anti-histamine).

II.
Side Effects: anxiety, brain fog, constipation, depression, diarrhea, dizziness, elevated blood pressure, fatigue, gastritis, hair loss, headache, hives (from Aimovig), indigestion, irregular heartbeat, jaw pain, kidney problems, low blood pressure, lower libido, mania, nausea, osteoporosis, ptosis (eyelid drooping from Botox), queasiness, rash, restlessness, Spock eyebrow (from Botox), stroke, tremors, ulcer, vascular events, vertigo, weight gain, weight loss, excessive daytime sleepiness, yellowing of eyes (liver malfunction), zinc deficiency.

Results: mixed. Conclusion: none—most days my migraine accompanies me.

Maiden, Mother, Crone

—text from advertisement for Lydia E. Pinkham's Vegetable
Compound (1938) in my great-grandmother's hometown
newspaper, *The Rolfe Arrow* (Rolfe, Iowa)

Do you feel so nervous you want to scream?
Are you cross and irritable?
Do you scold those dearest to you?
If your nerves are on edge,
try Lydia E. Pinkham's
Vegetable Compound
It often helps nature calm
quivering nerves.
For three generations
one woman has told another
how to go "smiling through"
with Lydia E. Pinkham's
Vegetable Compound.
It helps nature tone up the system,
thus lessening the discomforts
from the functional disorders
which women must endure.

Headache Stone

When the plates of my skull rumble and the earth shifts beneath my feet, I conjure the headache stone of Saint Áed, who entered this world marked for pain, having dashed his head on a rock at birth, his skull cleaving a hole into which rainwater falls, pooling in a little font. I lay my head in the central depression, place my elbow in the smaller divot—bone on stone—and pray for release.

****

A man who was suffering from a great pain in the head came to St. Áed and said: O holy man of

****

God I am very plagued by headache, and pray for me. The bishop said to him: In no way will

****

that pain depart from you, unless it will come over me: but you will gain great merit, if you bear

*****************************   ******************************
*****************************   ******************************
*****************************   ******************************
*****************************   ********* ****************
****************************   *********   ****************
***************************   ********* ****************
****************************   ******************************
****************************   ******************************
****************************   ******************************
******************************   ***************************
****

it patiently. He answered, Sir, the pain is beyond my forces. St. Áed said: the pain in your head

****

O Man may come into my head. And immediately the pain descended into the Bishop's head and

****

that man went out healthy and giving thanks. – Acta Sanctorum Hiberniae, John Colgan (1645)

****

Incantation

Head of Eva,

eye of Mary, forehead of Irene,

nose of Sarah, lips of Ann,

tongue of Bridget, neck of Nellie,

mind of Margaret, heart of Eleanor,

grace of Lovisa, faith of Ruth

blood of Magdalena.

Great-, great-, great-grandmothers,

mothers, daughters—

Amen

This is chanted every time my head blazes. After I say their names, I place my head in my palms and rub my temples, massage my forehead. I say three Hail Marys because I want my mother, my grandmothers— the ones who understand. I know they would take my pain into their bodies if they could, just as I would for my daughter. We can't. I ask for their strength, imagine a laying on of cool maternal hands.

Self-Portrait as Warming Planet

I felt a funeral, in my brain...

—Emily Dickinson

The sky burns from the top
down, ocean a churn of cinders.

My brow molten, I hiss, spitting
lava into smoking sea.

Singed feathers float. Which way
is up? Fish gasp, dolphins pant. I flush,

sweat, cry. Don't even try to deny it.
Once a friend wrote *I can make a bird*

fly out of your mouth backwards. I wish
I could put things in reverse.

My ovaries are misfiring,
brain aflame. Is it still a menstrual

migraine if you no longer bleed?
My skin cracks. It's *the end of pink,*

of green, fields barren, dry.
Soon I'll be invisible.

Mums

...a thirteen-year-old with the experience and daily life of a forty-five-year-old.

—Mary Ruefle, "Pause"

Hardy or not, the mums have had it, battered
by October snow and cold even today's bright

warmth can't undo. Faces downcast, shriveled heads
droop on broken necks, brittle roots digging heels

into dry dirt, struggling for a foot hold, too late—
they've lost too much ground to recover their youth.

I lean closer, peer with presbyopic eyes at purple jewel
tones faded to a muted mauve, watercolor tresses

streaked gray. The dog pees on them, adding insult
to injury. They shrug in surrender. The gaggle of flower

crones tilts bladed crowns toward me, so many petaled
ears ready for secrets to be shared before their balding

skulls are fully sheared. The truth: sometimes I scream
and curse at my children inside my head, inside my house.

Especially the girls—it's like looking in the mirror.
I wouldn't say hate but I would say rage. A whole roiling

tank of it, the saltwater cavity where my darlings grew
now filled with hormonal sludge, source of *abnormal*

bleeding to be explored by ultrasound. Last night's dream
flashes back—scrubbing filthy toilets, taking out trash

bags, bloody paper towels glaring through white plastic,
snatches of the murder mystery I was watching in bed

subsumed in the brain's slag heap: another female body
brutalized on the bathroom floor.

The Fathers of Modern Headache Medicine Discuss
the Migrainous Woman and All Her Troubles

—Dr. Harold G. Wolff and Dr. Walter C. Alvarez, as quoted in
newspapers and other publications (1945-1949)

I can often recognize the migrainous woman
the minute I see her; this is very helpful

diagnostically, because often she is rather sensitive
about her handicap. Most of these women tend

to be petite and with nice (full-breasted) figures.
They are usually above average in intelligence

and social charm. They are tense, quick
in understanding and in movement. They are idealistic,

wanting perfection. They want things done fast,
and "just so." They are unusually sensitive to noises,

bright lights, and unpleasant odors. They faint
and fatigue quickly under strain and excitement.

They get so tense over thinking of doing something
that they can get a headache even before they get started.

The outstanding characteristics of the migrainous
woman are her hypersensitiveness and tendency to worry,

to tire easily, to wilt suddenly, to sleep poorly.
The migrainous woman is reluctant to accept

the consequences of maternity and may have a hard
myomatous uterus, a wandering womb. The exciting cause

of the attacks is marital infelicity. Orgasm is seldom
attained and the sex act is accepted as, at best, a reasonable

marital duty. Migrainous women make a mess of their lives
because they customarily waste $10 worth of energy

on a ten-cent problem. The solution lies in talking over
her life problems and in showing her how to live

more calmly and happily because she isn't tough enough
or heartless enough to get the divorce she craves.

Migraine Disability Assessment Test Redux

It is an axiom with me that whenever a woman is having three attacks of migraine a week, it means that she is either psychopathic or else she is overworking or worrying or fretting or otherwise using her brain wrongly.

—Dr. Walter C. Alvarez (1945)

The Migraine Disability Assessment Test

question ▒▒▒ your
headaches ▒▒▒ your life ▒▒▒ help ▒▒▒ primary care provider
treatme▒▒▒

INSTRUCTIONS

Please ▒▒▒

▒▒▒ Please ▒▒▒ healthcare professional.

_____ 1. ▒▒▒ your headaches?

_____ 2. ▒▒▒ your headaches? ▒▒▒

_____ 3. ▒▒▒ your headaches?

_____ 4. ▒▒▒ your headaches? ▒▒▒

_____ 5. ▒▒▒ your headaches?

_____ ▒▒▒

What you ▒▒▒ **need to know** ▒▒▒:

_____ A. ▒▒▒ many days ▒▒▒ you have a headache ▒▒▒ each day ▒▒▒

_____ B. ▒▒▒ painful ▒▒▒ headaches ▒▒▒ pain ▒▒▒ pain ▒▒▒

Scoring: ▒▒▒ you ▒▒▒ question ▒▒▒ gnore ▒▒▒

▒▒▒	▒▒▒	▒▒▒
▒	▒▒▒ Disability	▒▒
▒	Mild ▒▒▒	▒▒
▒	Moderate ▒▒▒	▒▒
▒	Severe ▒▒▒	▒▒

▒▒▒ **please** ▒▒▒ **doctor** ▒

Faith Healing

O barefoot nun, Doctor
of the Church,
do you remember me?

Teresa, I made a pilgrimage
to your city of toothed walls,
knelt to venerate
your twisted finger
in its glittering reliquary.

O Patron, Sister,
if you can't take away my pain,
I understand—
but send me a sign
that you believe:

reach out your shriveled
holy hand
so your faith
can heal me.

Postdrome

*For when the pain recedes, ten or twelve hours later, everything goes with it,
all the hidden resentments, all the vain anxieties. The migraine has acted as a
circuit breaker, and the fuses have emerged intact. There is a pleasant
convalescent euphoria.*

—Joan Didion, "In Bed" (1968)

Oh, to hibernate
like an animal in a cave,
to curl nose to tail
in humid darkness,
lulled by water
dripping on stone.

To sleep for hours
as if day were night,
to recline, supine
like a corpse laid out flat,
tucked under cool sheets
pulled up to my chin, lips ajar—
sweet, sepulchral slumber.

And finally, to rise
languid as honey,
opening heavy-lidded eyes
to find the world shiny
but not too bright:
a waking dream that unfurls
in cerulean, gold and green.

Ode to the Jaw

This is for the twin hinge,
hardest of bony workers,
gatekeeper of body and mind,
guardian of the toothed cave,
vestibule for breath and sustenance.
Puppeteer behind the scenes,
you crank the red drawbridge,
sheriff of the mouth,
keeper of speech, teacher of suck
and kiss, damp-lipped clamp.

Is it any wonder you yawn
and ache? You are Sisyphus
of swallowing, Atlas of the palate,
tamer of muscular
tongue and teeth. You are chewer
of words and meat, mandible
and maxilla in marriage
of opposites, chomping till death
do you part: holy equation of catch
and release. You are holder of tension,
detritus of language, emotion
ground down by the tectonics
of the molar ridge. Tender buttons,
jointed joist of bone on bone,
clenched or unseated in sleep
you rouse the three-headed dragon,
trigeminal and terrible, to unleash
a shower of darts shimmering
from eye socket to cheek.

O simple machine, mother
who feeds, domed cathedral
of want and need. O
sacred portal that falls open
at rest when the soul is released.

Self-Portrait at 45, on the Autumnal Equinox

(Northern Hemisphere)

And the sugar maple (}
is already touched (}
in the head, red
around the edges. (}
Last night, death grasped
a handful of scalloped green
to press to cold lips in a kiss, (}
sucking all the blood,
from the heart—
rivers of vermillion }
rising through capillaries
to the surface. Today,
celestial scales balance {)
darkness and light.
Brilliant bruises blaze ( )
at tips of branches,
bleeding extremities
that will spread {)
before they peak
and fade. {)

Notes

Migraine is the third most common disease in the world, affecting one in seven people globally, and three times as many women as men (American Migraine Foundation). The text for the found poems comes from newspaper articles about migraine and advertisements for headache remedies from the time (1896-1961) and places (small, rural towns in Indiana and Iowa) where my great-grandmother—who experienced hemiplegic migraines that caused one-sided, temporary paralysis—lived.

The epigraph for "Annunciation" is a quote by German Benedictine abbess, scientist, composer, mystic, and healer Hildegard of Bingen from her illuminated text, *Scivias* (1152), which contains writings and illustrations of her visions that some scholars believe depict migraine aura, a claim rejected by medical historian Katherine Foxhall in her book, *Migraine: A History* (2019). Hildegard also wrote several texts (*Physica*, *Causae et Curae*) containing remedies for illnesses and injuries. The poem incorporates (italicized) lines from Luke 1:38 and alludes to Matthew 26:39. The image of my "head exploding" is borrowed from Cynthia Marie Hoffman (also a migraineur), whose memoir-in-prose-poems about OCD is entitled *Exploding Head*.

"Migraine Disability Assessment Test 1" and "Migraine Disability Assessment Test Redux" are erasures of the MIDAS questionnaire published by AstraZeneca Pharmaceuticals (2007) and Innovative Medical Research (1997), which is used as a screener for migraine. The epigraph for "Migraine Disability Assessment Test" comes from a letter Hildegard of Bingen wrote describing her experience of the *umbra viventis lucis*, or "reflection of the living light."

The epigraph for the sonnet "Our Lady of the Burning Bush" comes from the Book of Exodus, Chapter 3, Verse 2 of the Bible, describing Moses' encounter with the burning bush on Mount Sinai. Our Lady of the Burning Bush (also known as the Theotokos or Virgin of the Unburnt Bush) is venerated in the Orthodox Church on September 4.

"Cortical Spreading Depression" describes the wave of altered brain activity that is hypothesized to underly the visual and sensory auras of migraine (and other neurological conditions, such as epilepsy). Once started, the process is difficult to abort. The event horizon of a black hole is the "point of no return:" a boundary that, once crossed, nothing, not even light, can escape.

The epigraph for "Revenant" is an incantation from section *Cranium 3* of *The Nineveh Medical Encyclopaedia* (c. 7th c. B.C.E.), a compendium of medicine recorded in cuneiform script on clay tablets at the Royal Library at Nineveh, translated in the online Open Richly Annotated Cuneiform Corpus (ORACC).

The text on the left side of "In Her/My Head" comes from the visit summary notes and discharge instructions written by the doctor who attended me at an urgent care clinic visit for a severe migraine episode. The epigraph is a quote from "On Being Ill" (1926) by Virginia Woolf.

"Remedia" is a found poem from *Bald's Leech Book* (c. 950 C.E.), a text of Anglo-Saxon remedies, as quoted in Katherine Foxhall's book, *Migraine: A History* (2019).

The italicized text in "Prayer for the Intercession of Saint Teresa of Ávila, Patron Saint of Migraines" comes from *Mrs. Corylon's Booke of Diuers Medecines, Broothes, Salues, Waters, Syroppes, and Oyntementes* (1607), an early modern household recipe book. Mrs. Corylon's *Booke* is quoted in Katherine Foxhall's book, *Migraine: A History* (2019). St. Teresa of Ávila is the patron saint of migraines and headaches in the Catholic Church.

The epigraph for "Photophobia" is the first line of "In a Dark Time" by Theodore Roethke.

"A Kind of Brainstorm" is a found visual and prose poem inspired by the "Ascertaining capacity of cranial cavity by means of water" photo series in the digital archive of the collections of the National Library of Medicine. The text of the poem comes from an article in *The Waterloo Press* (Waterloo, Indiana) November 6, 1913, entitled "What is Migraine."

The woman at the bottom of the poem, with the beehive-like updo echoing the misshapen skulls of the images, is my great-grandmother, Eva (1896-1961).

The text of the found poem, "On the Heredity of Migraine" comes from the following two columns: "Health Talks by William Brady, M.D., Noted Physician and Author. Questions and Answers," *Journal and Courier*, Lafayette, Indiana, February 3, 1921; and "Personal Health Service: The Aura of Migraine." *Cedar Rapids Gazette*, Cedar Rapids, Iowa, April 29, 1931.

"MRI" includes images and text from my own MRI.

"In Bed" borrows its title from Joan Didion's 1968 essay of the same name, which was reprinted in *The White Album*, Noonday Press, 1990.

The text for the found poem "Maiden, Mother, Crone" comes from an advertisement for Lydia E. Pinkham's Vegetable Compound in the *Rolfe Arrow*, Rolfe, Iowa, April 14, 1938. Rolfe is the town nearest the farm on which my great-grandmother lived during the time it was published.

The italicized text in "Headache Stone" describes St. Áed Mac Bricc (also called St. Hugh), a 6th century Irish saint and Bishop of Killare, and comes from the *Acta Sanctorum Hiberniae* (Acts of the Irish Saints) by John Colgan (1645). Saint Áed was said to have hit his head on a stone (which retained the mark) at his birth, thereby endowing him with the ability to cure headache. St. Áed's bullaun stone, a large rock with a central depression and a smaller one, is believed to relieve head-aches if a sufferer lays their head on it.

"Incantation" mirrors the structure of one of the *Saint Gall Incantations* from the Abbey of Saint Gall in Switzerland, c. 922-926 C.E. It incorporates the same form by blessing the body parts afflicted by headache but substitutes the names of my matrilineal ancestors, including my mother, grandmothers, and daughter. The text of the original incantation (of which there are various translations) and instructions follow:

Head of Christ, eye of Isaiah, forehead of Elijah, nose of Noah, lips of Job, tongue of Solomon, neck of Matthew, mind of Benjamin, heart of Paul, grace of John, faith of Abraham, blood of Abel, Holy, holy, holy Lord, Lord God Sabaoth. Amen. This is sung every day about thy head against headache. After singing it thou puttest thy spittle into thy palm and thou puttest it round thy two temples and on thy occiput, and therat thou singest thy paternoster thrice, and thou puttest a cross of thy spittle on the crown of thy head, and then thou makest this sign, U, on thy head.

The epigraph of "Self Portrait as Warming Planet" comes from Emily Dickinson's "I felt a Funeral, in my Brain, (340)." The line "the end of pink" is borrowed from Kathryn Nuernberger's poem from her collection, *The End of Pink*.

"Mums" includes an epigraph from Mary Ruefle's essay, "Pause," about menopause.

The text for "The Fathers of Modern Headache Medicine Discuss the Migrainous Woman and All Her Troubles" comes from two newspaper articles in which Dr. Walter C. Alvarez is quoted: "Beauty is a Headache," by Gobind Behari Lal, "Noted Science Analyst," in the *Pittsburgh Sun-Telegraph* February 18, 1945; and "Many Women Worry Themselves Sick, Says a Noted Mayo Doctor," By G.B. Lal, Science Editor, *The Atlanta Constitution* September 11, 1949. Additional quotes by Alvarez and Dr. Harold G. Wolff, including the title of Alvarez's paper, "The Migrainous Woman and All Her Troubles," come from the book *Not Tonight: Migraine and the Politics of Gender and Health* by Joanna Kempner (2014).

The epigraph for "Migraine Disability Assessment Test Redux" is a (1945) quote from Dr. Walter C. Alvarez, often regarded, along with Dr. Harold G. Wolff, as one of the 'founding fathers' of migraine treatment.

"Faith Healing" contains images of the shrine and relics of St. Teresa of Ávila in Spain. St. Teresa was named a Doctor of the Church, a title given to canonized saints who have made significant scholarly and theological contributions to Church doctrine and teachings. Of the 37 Doctors of the Catholic Church, only four are women; Hildegard of Bingen is also a Doctor of the Church.

"Postdrome" includes an epigraph from Joan Didion's essay "In Bed." The postdrome, sometimes called a migraine "hangover," is a period of fatigue, brain fog, and mood changes which can persist for hours or days.

Acknowledgments

I am grateful to the editors of the publications in which the following poems, sometimes in different versions, have appeared:

"Postdrome," *Capsule Stories* (originally titled Dysthymia)
"Faith Healing," *Cider Press Review*
"Migraineur," *Halfway Down the Stairs*
"Migraine Abecedarian," *Lunch Ticket–Amuse Bouche*
"Self-Portrait as Warming Planet," *Rogue Agent*
"Ode to the Jaw," *SWWIM*
"Our Lady of the Burning Bush" (originally titled "Self-Portrait with Migraine"), *Valparaiso Poetry Review*
"Mums," *West Trade Review*
"The Fathers of Modern Headache Medicine Discuss the Migrainous Woman and All Her Troubles," *West Trestle Review*

I also extend my heartfelt gratitude to the many people who helped bring this project to fruition:

To the editors at *Chestnut Review*, especially Maria S. Picone (migraine sister), whose care and insightful input brought these poems, and the arc of the manuscript, into sharper focus.

To visual artist Sheila "Shee" Gomes, who read my manuscript and painstakingly converted many MRI images of my brain to create a beautiful, personalized, and inspired cover design.

To Carolyn Oliver, for her editorial flourishes and friendship.

To my migraineur community of writers, who generously read and blurbed this manuscript: Cynthia Marie Hoffman, Rita Maria Martinez, and Sarah M. Sala.

To my neurology team, Dr. Gary Keilson, Kate Williams, and Carolyn Benson, for helping me manage my migraines and feel better.

To my teachers in the Pacific University MFA Program, especially Kwame Dawes, Dorianne Laux, and Joseph Millar.

To my writing kindreds Maureen Boyd, Kimberly Casey, Sarah Elkins, Tink Faulise, Mandy Gutmann-Gonzalez, Melissa McKinstry, Carolyn Oliver, Tina Posner, Sarah Sullivan, N. L. Shompole, Elizabeth Sylvia, and Jeanne Yu: your art inspires me; your friendship sustains me.

To my family, especially my husband, Ed, for their understanding and love.

To my mother, for her empathy and support.

To my great-grandmother, Eva, for surviving and thriving. This is for you.

About the Author

Therese Gleason is author of *Matrilineal* (Finishing Line, 2021), which received Honorable Mention for the Jean Pedrick Chapbook Prize from the New England Poetry Club, and *Libation*, selected by Kwame Dawes as co-winner of the 2006 South Carolina Poetry Initiative Chapbook Competition. Her poetry, fiction, and essays have appeared in *32 Poems, Cincinnati Review, Indiana Review, New Ohio Review, Rattle,* and elsewhere. An educator, she has an MA in English from the University of Kentucky and an MFA in Poetry from Pacific University. Therese has taught ESL, composition, and creative writing at the college level, and has worked as a certified dyslexia therapist and Spanish teacher for students in elementary and middle school. Originally from Louisville, Kentucky, she currently lives in central Massachusetts with her family, where she teaches English language and literacy to multilingual learners in a public elementary school. Find her online at theresegleason.com.

www.ingramcontent.com/pod-product-compliance
Lightning Source LLC
Chambersburg PA
CBHW030524130626
46549CB00007B/3088